D0151129

# Atlas of Laryngoscopy

Edited By

Robert Thayer Sataloff, MD, DMA
Mary Hawkshaw, RN, BSN, CORLN
Joseph R. Spiegel, MD, FACS

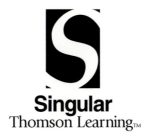

**Singular**
Thomson Learning™

8
RF514
.S28
2000

0411646937

**Singular Publishing Group**
**Thomson Learning**
401 West A Street, Suite 325
San Diego, California 92101–7904

**Singular Publishing Group** publishes textbooks, clinical manuals, clinical reference books, journals, videos, and multimedia materials on speech-language pathology, audiology, otorhinolaryngology, special education, early childhood, aging, occupational therapy, physical therapy, rehabilitation, counseling, mental health, and voice. For your convenience, our entire catalog can be accessed on our website at http://www.singpub.com. Our mission to provide you with materials to meet the daily challenges of the ever-changing health care/educational environment will remain on course if we are in touch with you. In that spirit, we welcome your feedback on our products. Please telephone (**1-800-521-8545**), fax (**1-800-774-8398**), or e-mail (singpub@singpub.com) your comments and requests to us.

© 2000, by Singular Publishing Group

Typeset in 10/12 Palatino by Flanagan's Publishing Services, Inc.

Printed in Canada by Transcontinental Printing

All rights, including that of translation, reserved. No part of this publication may be reproduced, stored in a retrieval system or transmitted in any form or by any means, electronic, mechanical, recording, or otherwise, without the prior written permission of the publisher.

**Library of Congress Cataloging-in-Publication Data**

Sataloff, Robert Thayer.
    Atlas of laryngoscopy / by Robert T. Sataloff, Mary Hawkshaw,
Joseph Spiegel.
        p.   cm.
    Includes index.
    ISBN 0–7693–0026–X (hardcover)
    1. Laryngoscopy Atlases.  2. Larynx—Radiography Atlases.
I. Hawkshaw, Mary.  II. Spiegel, Joseph Richard.  III. Title.
    [DNLM: 1. Laryngoscopy Atlases.  WV 17 S253a 2000]
RF514.S28  2000
616.2'2—dc21
DNLM/DNC
for Library of Congress
                                               99–33587
                                                CIP

# Contents

# Foreword

This *Atlas of Laryngoscopy* will be of great value, not only to practicing laryngologic surgeons, but also to residents in training, nurses, physicians in other specialties, medical students, voice therapists, and to patients who might have pathology similar to that described in this atlas. This tome is one of three separate volumes. The others are the *Atlas of Rhinoscopy* and the *Atlas of Otoscopy*. The endoscopic views in each atlas have appeared or will appear in the future as Clinics featured in the *Ear, Nose, and Throat Journal*.

When I accepted the position of Editor-in-Chief of the *Ear, Nose and Throat Journal*, I conceived the notion of including in each issue an endoscopic colored photography of the ear, nose, and throat accompanied by a brief description of the anatomy and pathology that was seen. The intent was not to provide a treatise of etiology, pathogenesis, and treatment, but rather to give a lesson to help the physician diagnose and understand what is seen.

The purpose was to entertain and to educate readers of the *Ear, Nose and Throat Journal*.

It has been a pleasure and my good fortune to work with Dr. Robert Sataloff and his colleagues who are experts in the field of voice and the larynx and who produce some of the world's best laryngoscopic pictures. Dr. Sataloff, who had a fellowship in neuro-otology, is also trained and very proficient in classical voice. He sings opera with perfection, which no doubt contributes to his empathy and special interest in the vocal folds. The first Laryngoscopic Clinic in the *Ear, Nose and Throat Journal* produced by Dr. Sataloff was published in Volume 72, Number 1, January 1993 and a clinic has been included every month since that time. This atlas provides a useful and lasting value for its owners.

Jack L. Pulec, MD
Editor-in-Chief
*Ear, Nose and Throat Journal*

# Preface

Although a small number of far-sighted professionals have been interested in the larynx and voice for centuries,[1] the field was not established as a subspecialty of otolaryngology until the 1980s. During the past 2 decades, there have been extraordinary advances in our understanding of the anatomy and physiology of phonation, vocal fold pathology, and in technology to visualize and quantify vocal fold structure and function. These advances have enhanced our understanding of vocal fold abnormalities, helping us understand the differences between nodules, polyps, cysts, and other structural abnormalities of the vocal folds.[2] Accurate differentiation between vocal fold pathologies is essential to plan optimal nonsurgical or surgical therapy.

As our ability to visualize and image vocal fold abnormalities improved, the differences between vocal fold lesions previously grouped as "nodules" or "polyps" became easier and easier to demonstrate. Because of growing interest among clinicians, in 1992, Dr. Jack Pulec, Editor-in-Chief of the *Ear, Nose and Throat Journal*, invited the author (RTS) to develop a monthly feature for this journal including a color photograph or video print and a discussion of an interesting vocal fold problem. The first article was published in January 1993. This atlas was developed because of comments by otolaryngologists on the usefulness of these Laryngoscopic Clinics in the *Ear, Nose and Throat Journal* by otolaryngologists and requests that they be compiled in a more convenient form. The atlas includes not only selected cases previously published in the Laryngoscopic Clinic feature section of the *Ear, Nose and Throat Journal*, but also numerous images and cases not published heretofore.

They are grouped roughly by diagnosis and are designed to show interesting features of many of the more common and clinically important vocal fold abnormalities seen by practicing otolaryngologists. We believe the images depicting vascular abnormalities of the vocal folds such as varicosities, ecstasias, and hemorrhages are particularly important because they have been traditionally underappreciated, frequently overlooked, and because their diagnosis and management is so important in achieving good long-term voice results for many patients with dysphonia, with or without concurrent vocal fold masses.

The authors hope that this atlas will prove interesting and useful for students, nurses, residents, fellows, speech-language pathologists, voice teachers, practicing otolaryngologists, and any other professional interested in vocal function and dysfunction and especially, in the structural abnormalities of the vocal folds.

Robert Thayer Sataloff, MD, DMA
Mary Hawkshaw, RN, BSN, CORLN
Joseph R. Spiegel, MD, FACS

## References

1. von Leden HA. A cultural history of the larynx and voice. In: Sataloff RT, *Professional Voice: The Science and Art of Clinical Care*. 2nd ed. San Diego, Calif: Singular Publishing Group; 1997:7–86.
2. Sataloff RT. Structural abnormalities of the larynx. In: Sataloff RT, *Professional Voice: The Science and Art of Clinical Care*. 2nd ed. San Diego, Calif: Singular Publishing Group; 1997:509–559.

**Joseph R. Spiegel, MD, FACS** is a graduate of Pennsylvania State University and Jefferson Medical College. He received training in general surgery at the Medical University of South Carolina in Charleston and completed residency in Otolaryngology—Head and Neck Surgery at the University of Michigan. Dr. Spiegel is an Associate Professor of Otolaryngology—Head and Neck Surgery at Thomas Jefferson University and Vice-Chairman of Otolaryngology—Head and Neck Surgery at Graduate Hospital. He has been in practice at 1721 Pine Street in Philadelphia since 1985.

# Contributors

**Mona Abaza, MD**
Assistant Professor of Otolaryngology—Head and
　Neck Surgery
University of Colorado
Denver, Colorado

**Nabil A. Abaza, DMD, PhD**
Professor of Oral and Maxillofacial Surgery and
　Pathology
Department of Surgery
MCP-Hahnemann School of Medicine
Philadelphia, Pennsylvania

**Margaret M. Baroody, MM, BS**
Singing Voice Specialist
American Institute of Voice and Ear Research
Philadelphia, Pennsylvania

**Carole Dean, MD, FRCS (C), CSPA**
Instructor
Department of Otolaryngology—Head and Neck
　Surgery
Thomas Jefferson University
Philadelphia, Pennsylvania
Fellow
American Institute for Voice and Ear Research
Philadelphia, Pennsylvania

**Kate A. Emerich, BM, MS, CCC-SLP**
Voice Pathologist
Wilbur James Gould Voice Research Center
Denver, Colorado

**Mary Hawkshaw, RN, BSN, CORLN**
Otolaryngologic Nurse Clinician
American Institute for Voice and Ear Research
Philadelphia, Pennsylvania

**Reinhardt J. Heuer, PhD**
Senior Research Scientist
American Institute for Voice and Ear Research
Philadelphia, Pennsylvania

**Cheryl A. Hoover, DMA, PA-C**
Physician Assistant
The Rochester Otolaryngology Group, PC
Rochester, New York

**Karla Kelleher, RN, MSN, CRNP, CORLN**
Otolaryngologic Nurse Clinician
American Institute for Voice and Ear Research
Philadelphia, Pennsylvania

**Karen M. Lyons, MD**
Clinical Assistant Professor of
　Otorhinolaryngology
Thomas Jefferson University
Philadelphia, Pennsylvania

**Amy Markiewicz, RN, BSN, CORLN**
Otolaryngologic Nurse Clinician
Executive Director of the American Institute for
　Voice and Ear Research
Philadelphia, Pennsylvania

**Anne A. McCarter, MD**
Otolaryngologist
Philadelphia, Pennsylvania

**Ron L. Moses, MD**
Clinical Instructor of Otolaryngology
Baylor College of Medicine
Attending Otolaryngologist
St. Luke's Episcopal Hospital
Houston, Texas

**Matthew Nagorsky, MD, FACS**
Department of Otolaryngology—Head and Neck
　Surgery
Graduate Hospital
Philadelphia, Pennsylvania

**Janette Ressue, MS, CCC-SLP**
Speech-Language Pathologist
Minneapolis, Minnesota

**Clark Rosen, MD**
Assistant Professor
Department of Otolaryngology—Head and Neck
　Surgery
University of Pittsburgh
Pittsburgh, Pennsylvania

**Deborah C. Rosen, RN, PhD**
Medical Psychologist
Bala Cynwyd, Pennsylvania

**J. Brian Same, MD**
Buffalo Otolaryngology Group
Buffalo, New York

**Dahlia M. Sataloff, MD, FACS**
Clinical Associate Professor of Surgery
The University of Pennsylvania
Attending Surgeon
Pennsylvania Hospital
Philadelphia, Pennsylvania

Ro

Pr

De

Th
Ch

Gr
Ad
Un
Ad
Ge
Ch
Th
Ph

# SECTION I

# Normal Vocal Folds

1    **Normal Anatomy of the Vocal Folds**
*Robert Thayer Sataloff*

# 1

# Normal Anatomy of the Vocal Folds

Robert Thayer Sataloff

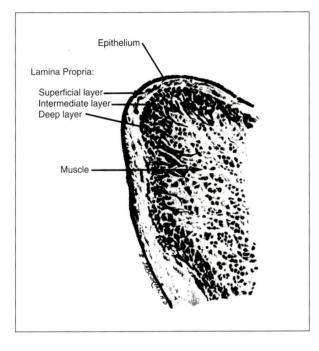

**Fig 1–1.** Layers of the vibratory margin of the vocal folds showing the epithelium; superficial, intermediate, and deep layers of the lamina propria; and vocalis muscle.

Despite centuries of fascination with the human voice, 20 years ago its structure and function were still not well understood. Scientific and technological advances during the last 2 decades have dramatically altered the standard of clinical voice care.[1-4] The availability of clinically practical slow motion assessment of the vibratory margin through strobovideolaryngoscopy has been particularly important. This technique permits everyday physical examination of the complex motions of the vocal fold edge. Interpreting videotaped stroboscopic evaluations requires familiarity with microscopic anatomy of the larynx, as well as considerable training and skill.

The soft tissue lining the larynx is much more complex than we had recognized until 1975 when Minoru Hirano described the layers of the vocal

fold.[5] The mucosa forms the thin, lubricated surface of the vocal folds that makes contact when they are closed. Interestingly, although most of the mucosa lining the larynx is pseudostratified, ciliated columnar (respiratory epithelium), the contact surfaces of the vocal fold are lined with stratified squamous epithelium, which is better suited to withstand the trauma of vocal fold contact.

The vocal fold is not simple muscle covered with mucosa. Beneath the epithelium lie the superficial, intermediate, and deep layers of the lamina propria and the thyroarytenoid (vocalis) muscle (Fig 1–1). The mucosa is connected to the superficial layer of the lamina propria through a basement membrane with extremely sophisticated architecture.[6] The 5 layers have different mechanical properties that are necessary to produce the smooth, shearing motions essential to healthy vocal fold vibrations (Fig 1–2).[1,7] Although the integrity of these layers is difficult to assess under continuous light (Fig 1–3), stroboscopic assessment permits observation of vocal fold function (Fig 1–4). Appreciation of the normal vibratory motion allows us to recognize even subtle pathology that may alter the anatomy and function of the vibratory margin of the vocal fold.

## References

1. Sataloff RT. *Professional Voice: The Science and Art of Clinical Care.* New York, NY: Raven Press; 1991.
2. Sataloff RT. The human voice. *Scientific American.* 1992; 267(6):108–115.
3. Gould WJ, Sataloff RT, Spiegel JR. *Voice Surgery.* Chicago, Ill: CV Mosby; 1993.
4. Sundberg J. *The Science of the Singing Voice.* DeKalb, Ill: Northern Illinois University Press; 1987.
5. Hirano M. Phonosurgery: basic and clinical investigations. *Otolagia (Fukuoka).* 1975;21:239–422.
6. Gray SD. Basement membrane zone injury in vocal nodules. In: Gauffin F, Hammarberg B, eds. *Acoustic, Perceptual, and Physiologic Aspects of Voice Mechanisms.* San Diego, Calif: Singular Publishing Group; 1991:21–27.
7. Hirano M. *Clinical Examination of the Voice.* New York, NY: Springer-Verlag; 1981:43–65.

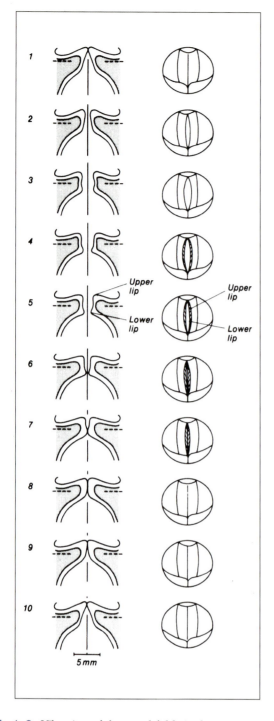

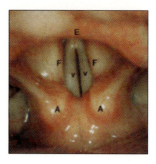

**Fig 1–3.** Photograph of the larynx under continuous light showing the vocal folds (V), false vocal folds (F), epiglottis (E), and arytenoids (A).

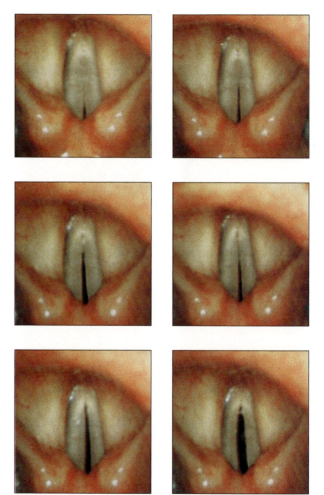

**Fig 1–2.** Vibration of the vocal folds is shown in a vertical cross section through the middle part of the vocal folds during the production of a single sound. The perspective is from the front of the larynx. Just before separation, the vocal folds are convergent (1). The glottis opens and closes (2–6) revealing a vertical phase difference. The inferior aspect closes first (7), and opens first (9–10) as subglottic pressure increases.

**Fig 1–4.** Selections from a sequence of photographs under stroboscopic light (Bruel and Kjaer, type 4914) illustrating the pattern of glottal opening from posterior to anterior.

# SECTION II

# Mucosal Abnormalities

# 2

# Gastroesophageal Reflux Laryngitis

Robert Thayer Sataloff
Joseph R. Spiegel
Mary Hawkshaw
Deborah C. Rosen

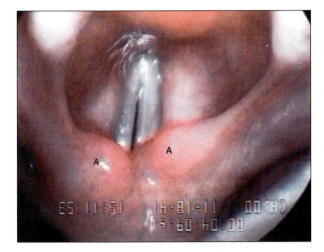

**Fig 2–1.** Normal larynx. Note that the mucosa overlying the arytenoids (A) is fairly similar in color to the mucosa lining other supraglottic structures.

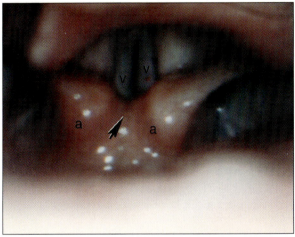

**Fig 2–2.** The typical appearance of reflux laryngitis. The arytenoids (a) and posterior laryngeal mucosa (arrow) are erythematous. The vocal folds (v) are within normal limits.

Gastroesophageal reflux is a condition caused by reflux of gastric contents into the throat. The condition has been well recognized for many years, and it has been associated with a variety of problems including hoarseness, sore throat, chronic cough, sensation of lump in the throat, halitosis, laryngeal granulomas, carcinoma of the esophagus and larynx, and others.[1-21]

Reflux laryngitis is extremely common. It has been reported in as many as 45% of professional voice users who seek medical care,[22] although it is often diagnosed incidentally and is not necessarily responsible for the patient's primary voice complaint. The diagnosis is often missed because of the absence of heartburn. In fact, classic dyspepsia is typically absent in patients with reflux severe enough to involve the vocal folds. Chronic sore throat (especially in the morning), morning hoarseness, excessive phlegm, minor swallowing complaints, and nocturnal cough are much more common symptoms.

Physical findings in patients with reflux laryngitis are consistent, although not pathognomic. Mild erythema of the pharynx is often present, but the most classic sign is arytenoid erythema (Figs 2–1 and 2–2). This is often associated with edema. In some cases, the erythema and edema may involve the entire larynx. More typically, only the arytenoid involvement is obvious. When arytenoid erythema is caused by voice abuse and frequent throat clearing, there is usually corresponding edema at the base of the epiglottis. When arytenoid erythema is limited to the posterior aspect of the larynx, reflux is by far the most common cause.

Various tests may be used to confirm the diagnosis of reflux laryngitis. If barium swallow is used, water siphonage maneuver should be added. The traditional barium swallow frequently yields false-negative results. Currently, the best available test appears to be 24-hour pH monitoring with proximal and distal sensors. The sensors are mounted on a tube placed through the nose. They measure acid levels throughout a 24-hour period. It is essential for the patient to work, talk, exercise, and perform all other normal daily activities (including singing). The patient should keep a log of the activities and times so that symptoms and activities can be correlated with episodes of reflux.

At present, the main aspects of therapy are elevation of the head of the patient's bed, avoidance of eating for a few hours before sleep, antacids, and $H_2$ blockers. However, many questions remain unanswered about the long-term effects of such therapy and about the effects of pH-neutral reflux. These and related concerns, along with the recent availability of laparoscopic fundoplication, suggest the possibility that recommendations for management of reflux may change over the next few years, and it would not be surprising to see an increase in the percentage of reflux patients referred for definitive surgical therapy.

## References

1. Cherry J, Margulies S. Contact ulcer of the larynx. *Laryngoscope.* 1967(November):1937–1940.
2. Goldberg M, Noyek AM, Pritzker KPH. Laryngeal granuloma secondary to gastro-esophageal reflux. *J Otolarygol.* 1978;7(3):196–202.
3. Teisanu E, Hecioia D, Dimitriu T, et al. Tulburari faringolaringiene la bolnavii cu reflux gastroesofagian. *Otorinolaringologia.* 1978;23:279–286.
4. Sataloff R. Professional singers: the science and art of clinical care. *Am J Otolaryngol.* 1981;8:251–266.
5. Carrasco E, Larrain A, Galleguillos F, et al. Asma bronquial y reflujo gatroesofagico. *Rev Med Chile.* 1982;110:527–537.
6. Henry R, Mellis CM. Resolution of inspiratory stridor after fundoplication: case report. *Aust Paediatr J.* 1982;18:126–127.
7. Ward PH, Berci G. Observations of the pathogenesis of chronic non-specific pharyngitis and laryngitis. *Laryngoscope.* 1982;92:1377–1382.
8. Andrieu-Guitrancourt J, Dehesdin D, Le Luyer B, et al. Role du reflux gastro-oesophagien au Cours des Dyspnées Aiguës Récidivantes de l'Enfant. *Ann Oto-Laryg.* 1984;101:141–149.
9. Barish CF, Wu WC, Castell DO. Respiratory complications of gastroesophageal reflux. *Arch Int Med.* 1985;145:1882–1888.
10. Olson NR. The problem of gastroesophageal reflux. *Otolaryngol Clin North Am.* 1986;19:119–132.
11. Ossakow SJ, Elta G, Colturi T, et al. Esophageal reflux and dysmotility as the basis for persistent cervical symptoms. *Ann Otol Rhinol Laryngol.* 1987;96: 387–392.
12. Koufman JA, Wiener GJ, Wu WC, et al. Reflux laryngitis and its sequelae: the diagnostic role of ambulatory 24-hour pH monitoring. *J Voice.* 1988;2:78–89.
13. Morrison M. Is chronic gastroesophageal reflux a causative factor in glottic carcinoma? *Otolaryngol Head Neck Surg.* 1988;99:370–373.
14. Kuriloff DB, Chodosh P, Goldfarb R, et al. Detection of gastroesophageal reflux in the head and neck: the role of scintigraphy. *Ann Otol Rhinol Laryngol.* 1989; 98:74–80.
15. Lumpkin SMM, Bishop SG, Katz PO. Chronic dysphonia secondary to gastroesophageal reflux disease (GERD): diagnosis using simultaneous dual-probe prolonged pH monitoring. *J Voice.* 1989;3:351–355.
16. McNally PR, Maydonovitch CL, Prosek RA, et al. Evaluation of gastroesophageal reflux as a cause of idiopathic hoarseness. *Digest Dis Sci.* 1989;34: 1900–1904.
17. Miko TL. Peptic (contact ulcer) granuloma of the larynx. *J Clin Pathol.* 1989;42:800–804.
18. Wiener GJ, Koufman JA, Wu WC, and et al. Chronic hoarseness secondary to gastroesophageal reflux disease: documentation with 24-H ambulatory pH monitoring. *Am J Gastroenterol.* 1989;84(12):1503–1507.
19. Katz PO. Ambulatory esophageal and hypopharyngeal pH monitoring in patients with hoarseness. *Am J Gastroenterol.* 1990;85(1):38–40.
20. Sataloff RT. Reflux and other gastroenterologic conditions that may affect the voice. In: Sataloff RT, ed. *Professional Voice: The Science and Art of Clinical Care.* New York, NY: Raven Press Ltd; 1991:179–183.
21. Freeland AP, Ardran GM, Emrys-Roberts E. Globus hystericus and reflux oesophagitis. *J Laryngol Otol.* 1974;88(10):1025–1031.
22. Sataloff RT, Spiegel JR, Hawkshaw M. Strobovideolaryngoscopy: results and clinical values. *Ann Otol Rhinol Laryngol.* 1991;100:725–727.

# 3

# Acute Laryngitis

Joseph R. Spiegel
Mary Hawkshaw
Amy Markiewicz
Robert Thayer Sataloff

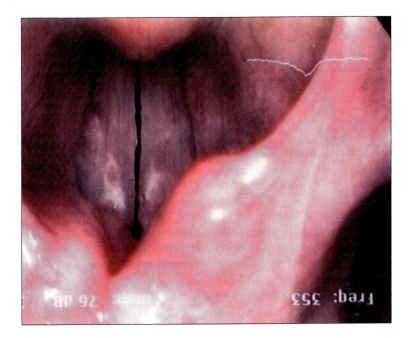

**Fig 3–1**

Following a recent performance, this 40-year-old classically trained operatic baritone complained of thick postnasal drainage and a feeling that his "cords were swollen." He had lifelong seasonal allergies but denied a recent increase in allergic symptoms. Strobovideolaryngoscopy (Fig 3–1) revealed acute laryngitis with erythema and edema of both vocal folds, copious thick secretions, and slight irregularities of both vocal fold edges. He also had other signs and symptoms of upper respiratory infection. His vocal folds and voice returned to normal following hydration, antibiotics, and relative voice rest.

# 6

# Prolonged Ulcerative Laryngitis

Joseph R. Spiegel
Robert Thayer Sataloff
Mary Hawkshaw

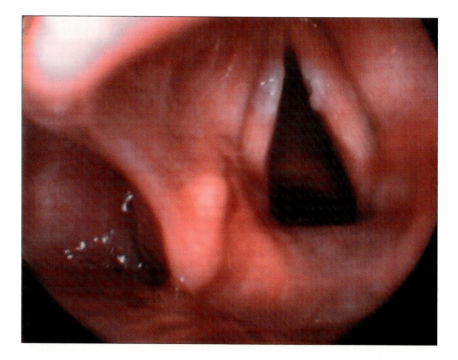

**Fig 6–1**

This 35-year-old music teacher in the public school system was trained as a professional singer, but she only uses her voice professionally in a classroom situation. She was a lifelong nonsmoker and nondrinker and had been treated in the past for gastroesophageal reflux disease. She presented after a 2-year absence from our practice with complaints of hoarseness, harsh cough, sore throat, and fever. Laryngeal examination revealed very edematous, mobile vocal folds with small nodular swellings and evidence of early laryngotracheitis. Initial treatment included Amoxicillin, a Medrol dosepak, voice rest, continued use of her Proventil inhaler, and Robitussin as needed for cough. She was seen 1 week later in the office in follow-up. At that time, her voice had remained hoarse, and she had a persistent cough and generalized fatigue Strobovideolaryngoscopy revealed severe vocal fold inflammation and ulceration, especially on the right vocal fold (Fig 6–1). She was then placed on a 10-day course of Biaxin, Prednisone, and complete voice rest. She was seen weekly in the office and ultimately received slightly more than 1 month's treatment with Biaxin, steroids, and vocal rest.

This case study was chosen to illustrate the nature of prolonged ulcerative laryngitis (PUL). This condition requires diligent surveillance and patience, as recovery time has been found to take from several weeks up to several months from the time of presentation. This patient's voice and vocal fold appearance returned to normal.

# SECTION III

# Vascular Abnormalities and Related Conditions

# 8

# Acute Vocal Fold Hemorrhage With Minimal Dysphonia

Robert Thayer Sataloff
Mary Hawkshaw
Deborah C. Rosen
Joseph R. Spiegel

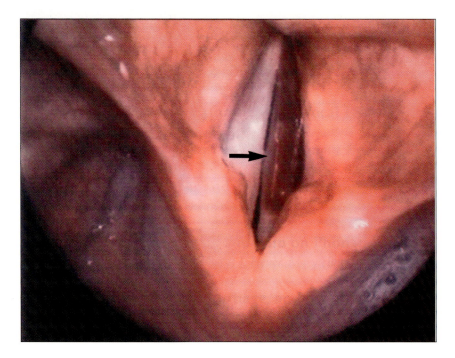

**Fig 8–1**

This 36-year-old police officer was struck in the larynx during an altercation. He was admitted to the hospital because of other injuries. Because of his history of laryngeal injury and mild hoarseness, direct laryngoscopy was performed promptly. He had a hematoma involving the superior surface of his right vocal fold (Fig 8–1).

Strobovideolaryngoscopy revealed that the vibratory margin was spared (arrow). This explains why the vocal fold looked so much worse than the voice sounded. Within 1 week, the vocal fold was flat (Fig 8–2), although still discolored. When the bulk of the hematoma resolves in this fashion, complete recovery generally occurs, as it did in this case. If a large mass of submucosal blood persists for more than a few days, incision and evacuation of the clot should be considered.

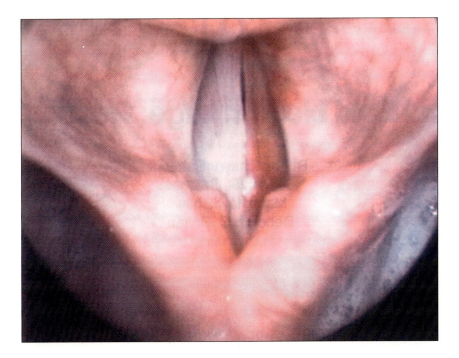

Fig 8–2

# 14

# Singing Dysfunction Following Vocal Fold Hemorrhage: The Need for Caution

Robert Thayer Sataloff
Joseph R. Spiegel
Reinhardt J. Heuer

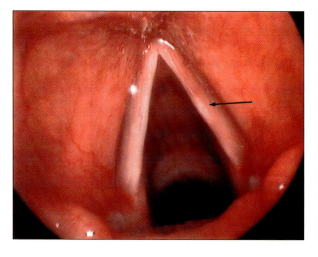

Fig 14–1

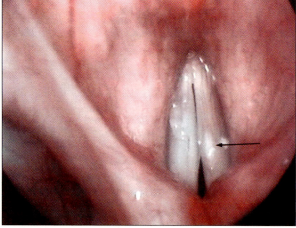

Fig 14–2

This 22-year-old woman had no voice problem until 6 months prior to evaluation. She had recently broken up with her boyfriend and was crying extensively when she developed sudden hoarseness, which got gradually worse over a 3-week period. She is not certain whether she was using aspirin or ibuprofen at the time, and she did not recall whether she was premenstrual when the voice change occurred. She is a trained singer and continued to perform despite her vocal fold hemorrhage. She was diagnosed as having bilateral vocal fold masses. Strobovideolaryngoscopic tapes were obtained from other laryngologists, and these observations were confirmed. When she came to Philadelphia for consultation, she had persistent hoarseness audible in her speaking voice, severe enough to interfere with her singing. Her singing technique was generally good. She had had no training for her speaking voice and demonstrated mild to moderate abusive

voice use. She aspired to an operatic career, and admitted to working as a restaurant hostess. She was in music school and also performed frequently. She had been advised to undergo excision of her persistent right vocal fold mass.

Strobovideolaryngoscopy revealed complete resolution of the left vocal fold mass. The videoprint above (Fig 14–1) shows a small persistent right vocal fold mass (arrow). However, more importantly, strobovideolaryngoscopy revealed stiffness throughout her entire edematous right vocal fold. The mass caused slight failure of glottic closure. Strobovideolaryngoscopy revealed clearly that most of her dysphonia was due to stiffness, rather than the mass. She was placed on relative voice rest, followed by intensive voice therapy (speech and singing). Her voice quality improved. So long as improvement continued, decisions regarding excision of the residual mass were deferred. However, once her voice stabilized, it was still unsatisfactory. Strobovideolaryngoscopy was used to determine that the mass was causing symptomatic failure of glottic closure (Fig 14–2). She underwent surgery, which resulted not only in elimination of the mass, but also in improvement in the mucosal wave. The operation was performed 11 months from the time of her original injury. She has enjoyed substantial voice improvement, glottic closure is complete, and she has resumed singing.

# 15

# Vocal Fold Varicosity Causing Voice Fatigue

Robert Thayer Sataloff

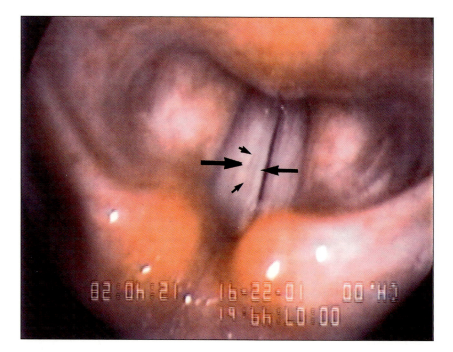

**Fig 15–1**

This 20-year-old conservatory voice major had been singing seriously for 5 years and had no voice problems until 10 months prior to examination. Initially, he noted voice fatigue and loss of his lower range after singing for approximately one-half hour. His voice problems became severe suddenly, during a concert, while he was trying to compensate for decreased volume and projection associated with voice fatigue. His voice remained hoarse for a week, after which his problems with rapid fatigue persisted. He admitted to symptoms of gastroesophageal reflux laryngitis. Comprehensive workup including laryngeal electromyography, with repetitive stimulation studies and appropriate blood studies, revealed no evidence of myasthenia or other neurological disorder.

The patient underwent strobovideolaryngoscopy on 2 occasions, 1 hour apart. The initial examination was normal. Immediately following examination he was taken to a piano and asked to sing until his voice fatigued. When fatigue occurred, strobovideolaryngoscopy was repeated, and the above videoprint was taken. It revealed a prominent varicosity on the left vocal fold. The large black arrow marks the lateral margin of the varicosity, the small arrow marks the medial margin, and the smallest arrow marks the anterior and posterior extent of the varicosity. This vein "pumped up" during singing, much as extremity veins become prominent during other forms of exercise. This added to the mass effect of the left vocal fold, causing interruptions in the vibratory pattern. Normal voice was restored by careful vaporization of the vessel.

# 16

# Varicosities and Vascular Masses

Robert Thayer Sataloff
J. Brian Same
Mary Hawkshaw

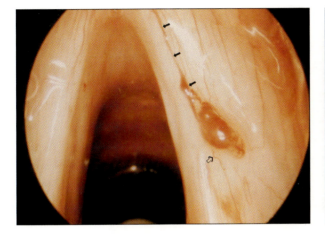

Fig 16–1

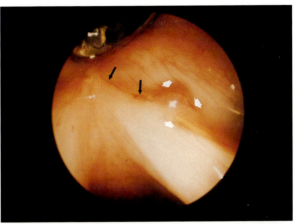

Fig 16–2

This 48-year-old singer, choir conductor, and orator had a 5- to 8-year history of hoarseness, an abnormal buzz in his lower range during speaking and singing, and complained of fullness and tenderness in his neck. A hemorrhagic vocal fold polyp was diagnosed by strobovideolaryngoscopy. Intraoperatively, he was found to have a large vascular polyp on the upper surface of the vibratory margin extending onto the superior surface on the right (Fig 16–1, 90° Storz telescope). This was contiguous with an abnormal and irregular vessel anteriorly (black arrows) and an irregular extension of the vessel posteriorly (open arrow). There was also a small punctate area on the left vibratory margin. Figure 16–2 shows the vascular mass (white arrows) with the vessel (black arrows) and left blush through a 70° Storz telescope. This provides a great deal more information about the topography of the lesion, and about the vessel anterior and posterior to the vascular mass on the right vocal fold. The patient underwent excision of his vascular mass, and dissection and excision of the aberrant vessel (as opposed to laser vaporization).

# 17

# Posthemorrhagic Vocal Fold Polyps

Robert Thayer Sataloff
Joseph R. Spiegel
Kate A. Emerich
Deborah C. Rosen

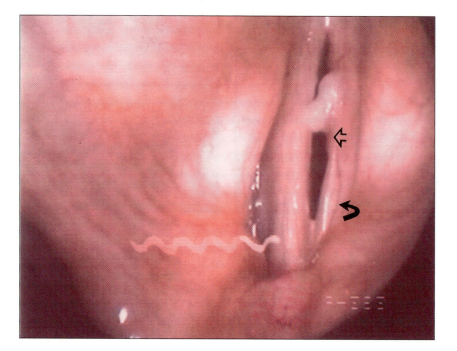

**Fig 17–1**

Vocal fold polyps are usually unilateral. They may be pedunculated or sessile. Although the etiology is often uncertain, in some cases, they clearly arise from vocal fold hemorrhage. This videoprint was taken during strobovideolaryngoscopy of a 67-year-old nonsmoker. He had noted hoarseness suddenly 1 month prior to this examination, and his dysphonia persisted. Strobovideolaryngoscopy revealed an irregular, varicose vessel along the superior surface of the right true vocal fold (curved arrow). The vessel loses its contour and disappears into a hemorrhagic blush near the base of the mass (open arrow). The bilobed, sessile, white polyp arising from the area still has areas of extravasated blood within it. Although medical management and voice therapy are generally worth trying for a brief period, such lesions ordinarily require surgery. Surgery should not only remove the mass, but also include cautious vaporization of the abnormal vessel, taking care not to injury the underlying vocal ligament.

# 18

# Symptomatic and Asymptomatic Hemorrhagic Cysts of the Vocal Folds

Robert Thayer Sataloff
Mary Hawkshaw
Karen M. Lyons
Joseph R. Spiegel

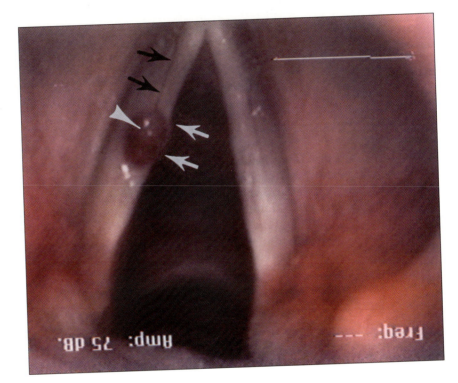

**Fig 18–1**

The consequences of vocal fold hemorrhage depend not only on completeness of resolution, but also on location. The 2 patients whose vocal folds are seen here have fairly similar lesions, but markedly different vocal consequences.

## Case 1

Case 1 is a 27-year-old professional singer who developed sudden hoarseness following a particularly taxing series of rehearsals, which preceded a scheduled recording session. Vocal fold hemor-rhage was diagnosed. The hemorrhage resolved partially, but a hemorrhagic cyst (Fig 18–1) per-sisted in association with an ectatic vessel (Fig 18–1, black arrows). This resulted in marked hoarseness and irregularity in the mid-range of her singing voice. Voice therapy eliminated her abusive com-pensatory gestures, but did not relieve her dyspho-nia. The lesion was removed surgically, and her symptoms resolved. Figure 18–1 also shows marked arytenoid erythema and posterior glottic pachyder-mia (partially visible at the bottom of the figure) caused by laryngopharyngeal reflux.

*Vascular Abnormalities and Related Conditions*

her right vocal fold (straight arrows). However, vocal fold vibration was normal, her voice was normal, and the varicosities appeared to have no functional effect. A diagnosis of atypical pain was made, and the patient was started on Tegretol. She stopped the medication because of planned pregnancy, and the pain returned. It resolved again when the Tegretol was resumed.

# 23

# Vocal Fold Cyst, Hemorrhage, and Scar in a Professional Singer

Robert Thayer Sataloff
Mary Hawkshaw

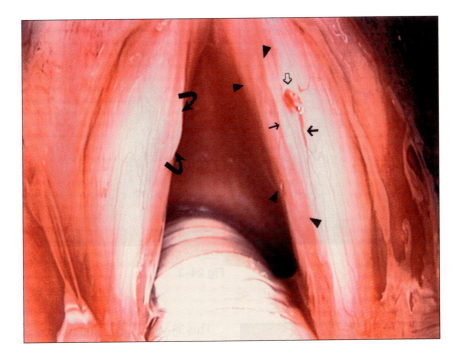

**Fig 23–1**

This 31-year-old professional soprano noted hoarseness while speaking following a demanding singing performance, which had been associated with vocal fatigue. Two days later, she developed sudden hoarseness while singing. Right vocal fold hemorrhage was diagnosed, and she was placed on voice rest. Hoarseness and vocal fold abnormalities persisted, and she was referred to our attention 3 months later. Her voice was soft, hoarse, and breathy.

Strobovideolaryngoscopy revealed right vocal fold scar consistent with previous hemorrhage, and the structural abnormalities seen on the intraoperative photograph (Fig 23-1). These include a left vocal fold cyst (curved arrows), right vocal fold varicosity (arrows) leading into an ectasia and post-hemorrhagic mass (open arrow), additional varicosities medial and lateral to the vascular mass, and diffuse scarring along the medial surface of the right vibratory margin (arrowheads). There was also a ridge of scar at the upper portion of the right vibratory margin (small arrow). Her masses and varicosities were excised, the scar was released, and the right vocal fold was medialized with autologous fat to improve glottic closure and ease of phonation. She had no recurrent hemorrhages or masses, but she had persistent stiffness of the right vibratory margin.

# SECTION IV

# Benign Lesions

# 28

# Vocal Fold Scar

Robert Thayer Sataloff
Joseph R. Spiegel
Mary Hawkshaw

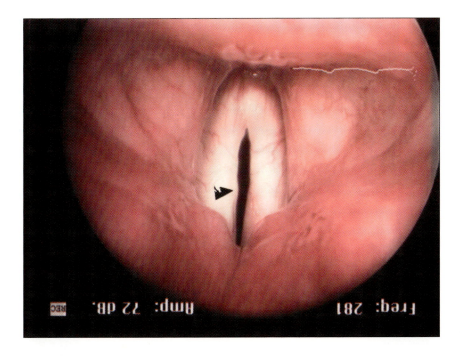

**Fig 28–1**

This 16-year-old former high school soprano soloist and cheerleader had no vocal problems until 18 months prior to evaluation when she gradually developed hoarseness over a period of 2 months. She was told that she had vocal nodules. No speech therapy was recommended nor provided. The "nodules" were removed by laser excision 1 year prior to our examination. She was essentially aphonic for 3 months following surgery and remained extremely hoarse, despite appropriate voice therapy. Strobovideolaryngoscopy (Fig 28–1) revealed severe bilateral vocal fold scarring and a small vocal fold mass (arrow). There was essentially no mucosal wave on the left, and the mucosal wave was markedly diminished on the right. Abnormal blood vessels running perpendicular to the vibratory margins are seen on the superior surface of both vocal folds. After another brief course of voice therapy, she underwent unilateral autologous fat implantation into the vibratory margin of the left (worse) vocal fold and excision of the mass. This resulted in improved glottic closure and return of a much improved mucosal wave. However, a second medialization procedure was required to achieve optimal voice quality.

# 31

# Chronic Voice Abuse and Bilateral Vocal Fold Cysts

Robert Thayer Sataloff
Mary Hawkshaw
Deborah C. Rosen
Joseph R. Spiegel

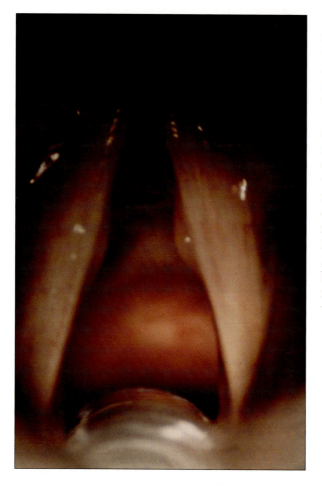

**Fig 31–1**

This 29-year-old woman is a high school mathematics teacher, aerobics instructor, sales representative, cheerleader, and cheerleading coach. She had a 5-year history of hoarseness. Her voice worsened following extensive use. She had previously been told she had vocal nodules.

Strobovideolaryngoscopy revealed bilateral, slightly asymmetric fluid-filled masses that deformed on contact. However, they were large enough to interfere with vibration and prevent glottic closure. The left mass was clearly a cyst. We were initially uncertain whether the right mass was a cyst or a soft, reactive nodule. Voice therapy resulted in no significant improvement. The videoprint on the left was taken at the time of microlaryngoscopy. At the time of surgery, both masses were found to be fluid-filled cysts. She healed well following resection of both masses, and her voice has been within normal limits for more than 1 year.

# 32

# Vocal Fold Cysts and Reactive Nodules: Differentiation From Bilateral Nodules

Robert Thayer Sataloff
Mary Hawkshaw
Joseph R. Spiegel
Cheryl Hoover

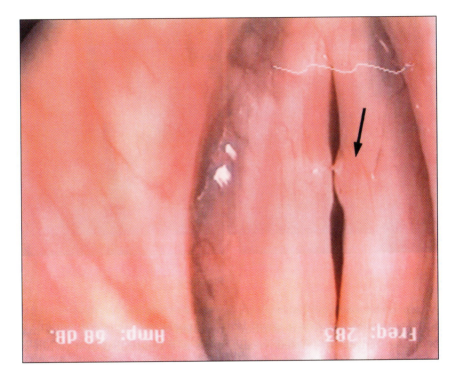

Fig 32–1

This 35-year-old stage and television actor developed hoarseness suddenly while acting. The role had extensive vocal and physical demands and required a particularly percussive vocal style and British accent. Review of strobovideolaryngoscopy performed by a physician who had treated him previously showed resolving hemorrhage in the right vocal fold with prominent vascularity on the superior surface of both vocal folds, as well as bilateral vocal fold masses. Our assessment was performed approximately 2 months following his original injury. Examination revealed a prominent blood vessel on the superior surface of the right vocal fold, running perpendicular to the vibratory margin (arrow) and leading into a fluid-filled submucosal cyst. There is a contact-induced nodule on the left vocal fold with a craterlike surface into which the right vocal fold cyst makes contact.

Expert voice therapy commonly results in resolution of contact nodules. However, cysts usually do not resolve through voice therapy alone. If a cyst remains symptomatic, surgical removal is appropriate. If therapy does not cure the contact nodule, surgical excision should also be considered. However, if the reactive nodule is soft to palpation at the time of surgery, it is reasonable to leave it undisturbed and observe the patient for resolution after the cyst has been excised.

# 37

# Vocal Fold Mass and Scar

Robert Thayer Sataloff
Anne A. McCarter
Mary Hawkshaw

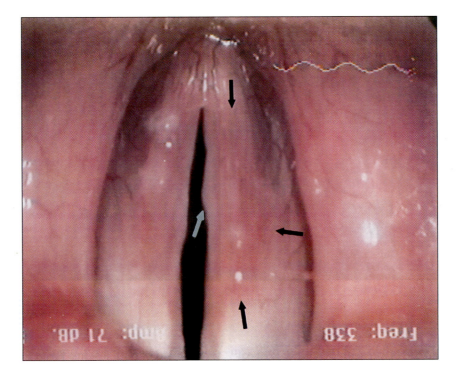

**Fig 37–1**

This 29-year-old alternative rock singer noted a voice change 9 months prior to evaluation while recording her first CD for a major label. She noted hoarseness at the end of each recording day during the course of her approximately month-long recording sessions. She had previously had a 4½-octave range. However, since the onset of her problems, her range had been reduced to 3 octaves. She had no concurrent illness and did not recall whether she was premenstrual at the time of her voice change. She was not using aspirin products. She had symptoms of reflux, which had not been diagnosed or treated at the time. Strobovideolaryngoscopy (Fig 37–1) showed a right vocal fold mass (white arrow), right vocal fold stiffness and scarring, a blush involving the scarred area (black arrows), left vocal fold stiffness, and a small left vocal fold mass. She underwent excision of her right vocal fold mass and medialization with autologous fat to help close the glottal gap caused by the vibratory margin stiffness. She has resumed her professional singing career.

# Vocal Fold Scar and Vocal Fold Nodules

Robert Thayer Sataloff
Joseph R. Spiegel
Deborah C. Rosen

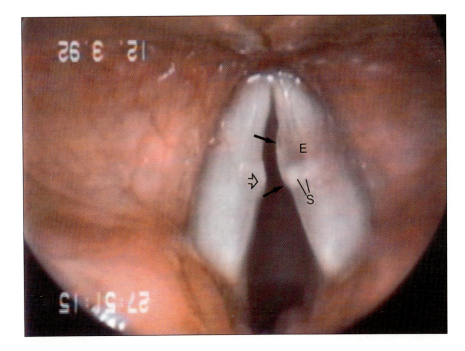

**Fig 38–1**

This 29-year-old woman first developed hoarseness during repeated episodes of screaming fights when she was 12 years old. She frequently went to school hoarse. Initially, her voice recovered. However, she also developed hoarseness after singing show music and in choirs. She became a professional dancer and singer. At approximately age 22, her hoarseness became persistent. A right vocal fold cyst was diagnosed and voice therapy was recommended by an excellent laryngologist in New York. She complied only briefly with that recommendation. For the following 7 years she remained constantly hoarse and noted inconsistency in the midrange of her singing voice and significant vocal fatigue after speaking or singing. Ten months prior to evaluation, her voice became much worse suddenly. Despite a successful career as an actress, dancer, and singer, she had begun voice training only shortly prior to our evaluation. Ongoing training and therapy had not produced improvement in voice quality.

Strobovideolaryngoscopy revealed bilateral vocal fold masses as illustrated in Figure 38-1. The right vocal fold mass (straight arrows) was broad-based, and it had a thick, deep white area of scar (S). There was also a broad area of slight discoloration (E) as is commonly seen following vocal fold hemorrhage. There was a solid, smaller white mass (open arrow) at the contact point on the left vocal fold. Strobovideolaryngoscopy revealed marked vibratory dysfunction on the right. These masses required surgical excision. However, because of the vibratory margin scarring, it was possible to predict preoperatively that a perfect result was unlikely.

# Vocal Fold Polyp, Scar, and Sulcus Vocalis

Robert Thayer Sataloff
Mary Hawkshaw
Matthew Nagorsky
Allyson Shaw

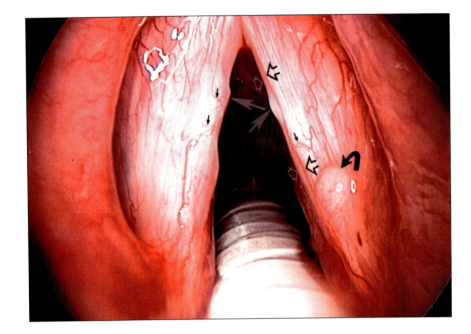

Fig 52–1

This 41-year-old female is a physical education teacher and a hockey, track, and basketball coach. She developed progressively worsening hoarseness over approximately 1 year. Seven months prior to our evaluation, she was diagnosed by another otolaryngologist as having vocal fold polyps. At that time, she underwent excision of both vocal fold masses. She had been placed on voice rest for 3 days. Her voice quality was worse following surgery. She had received no preoperative voice therapy. She had 4 sessions with a speech pathologist approximately 2 months following surgery, but she noted no improvement. She continued teaching, but found it difficult to do so because of hoarseness, decreased volume, and voice fatigue. She had a history of reflux, which had been treated in the past with Axid for 2 months. She had reflux symptoms but was on no medication at the time of our evaluation.

Strobovideolaryngoscopy revealed bilateral vocal fold scar with marked stiffness of the right vocal fold and essentially no vibratory motion of the left vocal fold. Following intensive voice therapy and reflux control, she underwent surgery. At the time of the operation (Fig 52–1), she was confirmed to have a polyp on the posterior superior surface of her right vocal fold (curved arrow), fibrotic masses on both vibratory margins (straight white arrows), right sulcus vocalis (open arrows), and numerous varicose vessels on the superior surfaces of her vocal folds, with aberrant vessels running toward (rather than parallel to) the vibratory margin, some of which are indicated by small black arrows.

She underwent staged surgery including fat implantation into her left vibratory margin, excision of her masses, and excision of the varicosities. She will probably require surgery for her right sulcus vocalis to optimize her phonatory result.

# 53

# Occult Mucosal Bridge of the Vocal Fold

Robert Thayer Sataloff
Clark Rosen
Mary Hawkshaw

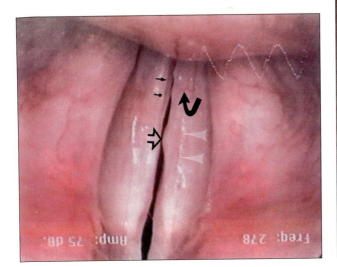

Fig 53–1

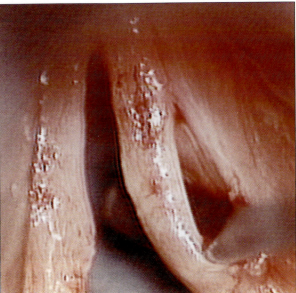

Fig 53–2

This 33-year-old singer and songwriter complained of dysphonia for 1 year, including hoarseness and loss of his high range. He had seen several otolaryngologists and had been treated with antibiotics, oral steroids, and inhaled steroids. At the time of our initial examination, he had severe erythema and thickening of his vocal folds, and his voice was hoarse. Steroids were stopped and he was treated for *Candida* laryngitis. The *Candidiasis* resolved. Numerous abnormalities were still present on strobovideolaryngoscopy after antifungal treatment (Fig 53–1). These included bilateral vocal fold stiffness, evidence of previous hemorrhage, left sulcus vocalis (Fig 53–1, small arrows), right vocal fold mass (Fig 53–1, open arrow), ectatic vessels on the superior surfaces of both vocal folds with a prominent vessel running at 90° to the vibratory margin (Fig 53–1, curved arrow), a small anterior glottic web, and muscular tension dysphonia. The importance of a line on the superior surface of the right vocal fold (Fig 53–1, white arrows) was not appreciated preoperatively. Intraoperatively, this was found to be the opening into an unusually large mucosal bridge (Fig 53–2). The mucosal bridge was removed, and autologous fat was injected laterally to medialize the right vocal fold and improve glottic closure.

# 60

# Endoscopic Internal Stent:
# A New Procedure for Laryngeal Webs
# in the Presence of Papilloma

Robert Thayer Sataloff
Mary Hawkshaw

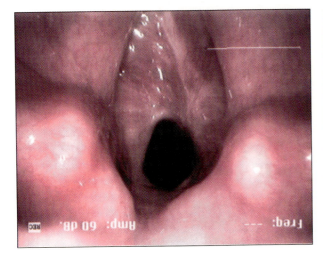

Fig 60–1

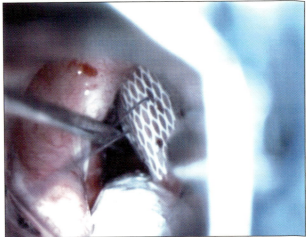

Fig 60–2

This professional speaker and businesswoman was 38 years old when we began caring for her in 1994. She had undergone resection of vocal fold masses in 1989 and in 1994, 9 months prior to our evaluation. She had an extensive papilloma involving the anterior commissure and both vocal folds and extending subglottally. There was a papillomatous web between the vocal folds. Resection of the anterior commissure papilloma involved division of the web; the left side was otherwise left undisturbed. Papillomas were resected from the right vocal fold, anterior commissure, and subglottic areas on December 19, 1994. In February 1995, she returned to the operating room for resection of the left vocal fold papilloma. She had already had extensive regrowth of her right papilloma and had reformed a web. In March 1995, she underwent division of the web and resection of the papilloma. All resections were performed with a combination of laser and cold instruments. She continued to have rapid, aggressive regrowth of papillomas. Surgery was performed only when symptoms were troublesome: in September 1996, November 1996, and January 1997. In all cases, extensive papilloma was resected from the glottic and subglottic areas above and below the recurrent web. Subglottic papillomas extended to the level of the cricoid cartilage. In March 1997, although only one vocal fold had been operated on at the time of her previous procedure, her web had enlarged and, for the first time, she had no gross evidence of papilloma. The web, however, interfered with her breathing. She returned to the operating room on March 12, 1997, at which time the web was divided and a flap was sutured superiorly on the left vocal fold and inferiorly on the right vocal fold. Because of her aggressive papillomatous disease, external surgery was avoided. We were concerned about

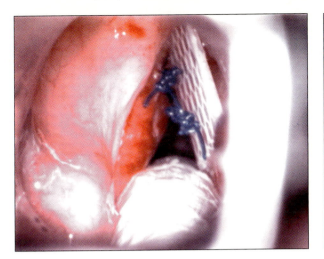

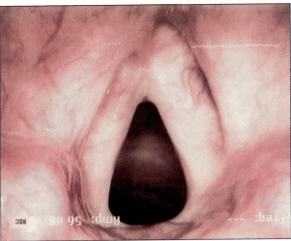

**Fig 60–3**

**Fig 60–4**

even passing sutures from the contaminated larynx to the skin, and we refrained from doing so. The web reformed promptly. It was divided bluntly 1 week following surgery. Because of the thickness of the web (approximately 6–8 mm in vertical dimension) and its extent (from, approximately, the vocal processes to the anterior commissure) (Fig 60–1), and because it was still producing respiratory symptoms, she returned to the operating room on April 12, 1997. To avoid the risks of transmitting papilloma to the skin, a new procedure was devised. Reinforced Silastic, 0.02 inches thick,

was sutured (Fig 60–2) endoscopically to the right vocal fold with Proline (Fig 60–3). The patient was followed as an outpatient until the left vocal fold appeared to be well mucosalized. She was returned to the operating room on the 26th postoperative day for stent removal. She has had reformation of a small web (Fig 60–4), which occurred within the first month, and has remained stable for 1 year. She has had no further airway difficulties. While she is still dysphonic, her voice is the best it has been for several years and is serviceable for social and business purposes. She has no evidence of papilloma.

# SECTION VII

# Leukoplakia and Keratosis

# 61

# Vocal Fold Masses Associated With Leukoplakia

Robert Thayer Sataloff
Joseph R. Spiegel
Mary Hawkshaw
Reinhardt J. Heuer

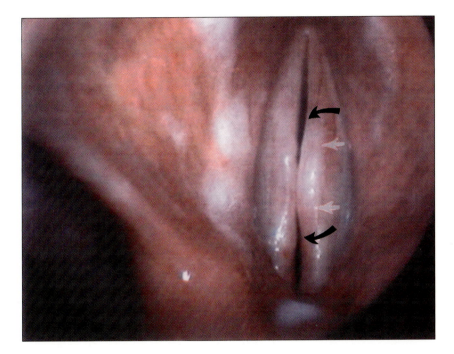

**Fig 61–1**

Some vocal fold masses cannot be diagnosed safely without prompt biopsy. This figure was taken during strobovideolaryngoscopy of an 82-year-old heavy smoker with a long history of hoarseness. He had been followed periodically by indirect laryngoscopy and had had no vocal fold masses until the time of this examination. Strobovideolaryngoscopy revealed a broad-based right vocal fold mass involving almost half of the right vocal fold. The curved arrows mark the anterior and posterior extents of the mass. The superior surface and vibratory margin have a broad white area (straight white arrows). The contact region of the left vocal fold revealed edema in Reinke's space and a questionable punctate hemorrhage posteriorly. Diffuse leukoplakia is also seen in the supraglottic area and posteriorly. Although there was no fixation of the mucosa, the epithelium was noted during strobovideolaryngoscopy to be somewhat thick and irregular. Biopsy was performed promptly when the lesions did not improve during a 4-week observation period accompanied by voice therapy and decreased smoking. The pathologist reported parakeratosis, mild dysplasia, viral-induced changes, and mild chronic inflammation with no evidence of acute inflammation or microorganisms. The changes were not typical of papilloma, viral cultures were unrevealing, and AFB stains were normal. The patient's voice returned to normal following excision of the mass and abnormal tissue. No biopsy was taken from the left vocal fold at the time of this procedure.

# 62

# Unusual Laryngeal Hyperkeratosis

Robert Thayer Sataloff
Joseph R. Spiegel
Deborah C. Rosen

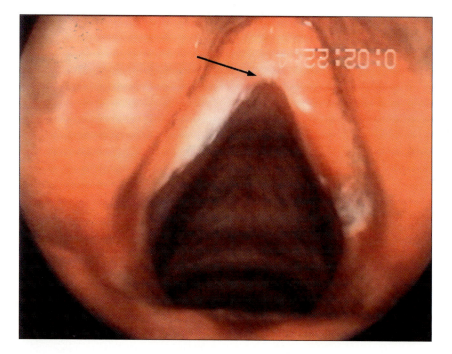

**Fig 62–1**

This 55-year-old man had a 2-year history of intermittent hoarseness. He had smoked 2 packs of cigarettes daily for 20 years, but had quit 16 years ago. He also had consumed large amounts of alcohol but had stopped drinking 6 years ago. Bilateral vocal fold leukoplakic lesions were excised by another otolaryngologist and found to be benign hyperkeratosis. He was referred for bilateral external auditory canal soft tissue occlusion. He underwent bilateral ear surgery for hyperkeratosis obliterans. At the time of initial examination, the patient had a small anterior web, no hyperkeratosis, and he reported that his voice was normal follow-ing surgery. Three years later, mild hoarseness and bilateral vocal fold hyperkeratosis recurred. The videoprint (Fig 62–1) above was taken at that time. Strobovideolaryngoscopy revealed an anterior glottic web (arrow), bilateral leukoplakia, prominent vasculature, and apparent thickening of the right vocal fold, but no evidence of fixation of the leuko-plakic lesions. Surgical excision revealed hyperker-atosis with no evidence of malignancy. There are no other areas of skin or mucosal abnormality, and it is uncertain whether the laryngeal hyperkeratosis and external auditory canal hyperkeratosis obliterans are causally related or coincidental.

# 63

# Vocal Fold Hyperkeratosis

Robert Thayer Sataloff
Mary Hawkshaw

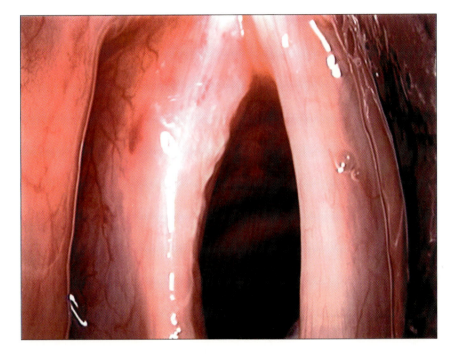

**Fig 63–1**

This 67-year-old physician and nonsmoker had had intermittent hoarseness for many years. However, for several months, his voice had been dysphonic most of the time. His voice was soft and hoarse, but he denied throat pain. He had no systemic complaints. He was unaware of reflux symptoms but admitted to excessive use of tabasco sauce. Strobovideolaryngoscopy revealed a thickened, irregular, partially leukoplakic lesion involving the anterior two thirds of the left musculomembranous vocal fold and extending onto the medial surface of the vibratory margin. The region of the abnormality was markedly hypodynamic under stroboscopic light. There were varicosities on the superior surface of the lesion, and prominent irregular vessels lateral to it. These findings were confirmed at the time of surgery (Fig 63–1). Submucosal infusion with saline and epinephrine was used at the time of excisional biopsy. Although the lesion was stiff, it was not fixed to the vocal ligament. The lesion was resected entirely without disturbing the surrounding noninvolved tissue. Histopathologic analysis revealed hyperkeratosis with intraepithelial atypia (dysplasia). He healed well and is being followed closely.

# SECTION VIII

# Carcinoma

This 71-year-(
our office 6 yea
At that time, he
ness. Examinati
Antireflux treat
hoarseness. He
ing the 6-year l
herence to anti
following his tr
heavily until 198
ing. He had a h
undergone antit
cal mycobacteri
intracellulari).

He returned a
cause of a 2-mor

# 65

# Squamous Cell Carcinoma of the Right Vocal Fold

Robert Thayer Sataloff

Joseph R. Spiegel

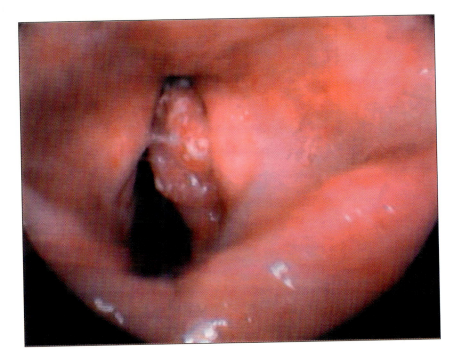

**Fig 65–1**

This 91-year-old man experienced sudden hoarseness 6 weeks prior to examination. He denied throat pain, otalgia, dysphagia, or weight loss, and he had no prior vocal difficulties. He had quit smoking 25 years prior to examination, following a 110 pack-year history, and he did not consume alcohol. Although cancer is not the most common cause of sudden hoarseness, it must always be considered in the differential diagnosis. The videoprint taken during strobovideolaryngoscopy revealed a $T_1N_0M_0$ squamous cell carcinoma. The exophytic mass involved the vibratory margin of the anterior two thirds of the right vocal fold, the anterior commissure, and extended across the midline to involve the interior 3 millimeters of the left vocal fold. There were 5 millimeters of infraglottic extension at the anterior commissure, but no subglottic extension more posteriorly. After computed tomography, he was treated with partial excision of the mass, followed by radiation therapy, consisting of 6,300 RADS. His voice improved substantially. He is still being followed closely.

# 66

# Vocal Fold Cancer Presenting as Sudden Dysphonia in the Absence of Risk Factors

Robert Thayer Sataloff
Mary Hawkshaw
Anne A. McCarter
Joseph R. Spiegel

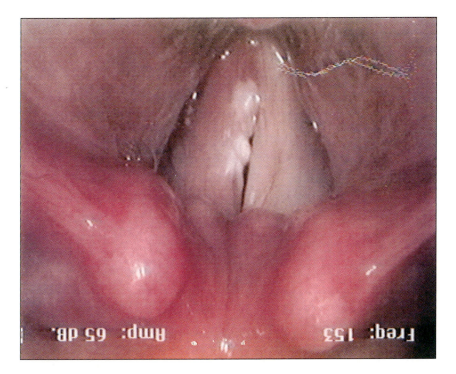

**Fig 66–1**

A 46-year-old voice teacher and performer had no vocal problems prior to a motor vehicle accident. Afterward, he reported that during the collision, he screamed loudly and that a seat belt had hit him across the front of the neck. He felt immediate hoarseness and throat pain. Three days after the accident, he sang two 30-minute performances. He found singing quite difficult vocally, and he had not performed since. He had had professional voice training since childhood, was a nonsmoker, and did not drink alcohol.

Strobovideolaryngoscopy revealed the presence of reflux laryngitis, left superior laryngeal nerve paresis, and a large bulky white mass on his left vocal fold (Fig 66–1). Laryngeal electromyography revealed mild paresis of both the left superior laryngeal nerve and the left recurrent laryngeal nerve.

Following objective voice measures and a brief course of voice therapy, microscopic direct laryngoscopy, and excisional biopsy were performed. Pathology revealed a squamous cell carcinoma of the vocal fold, which was classified as $T_3N_0M_0$. He was treated with radiation therapy. The sudden onset of dysphonia at the time of his motor vehicle accident remains unexplained, although we hypothesize that he may have hemorrhaged into his tumor. There was no evidence of injury to the other vocal fold.

# 67

# Anterior Laryngeal Transglottic Carcinoma

Robert Thayer Sataloff
Joseph R. Spiegel
Mary Hawkshaw
Deborah C. Rosen

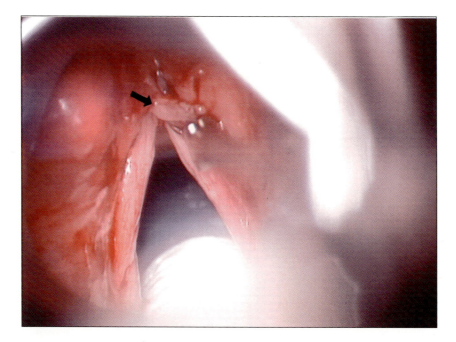

**Fig 67–1**

This 79-year-old woman had a 3-month history of hoarseness. She had smoked at least 1 pack of cigarettes daily for nearly 70 years. She had no history of throat pain or otalgia, and she denied dysphagia. The intraoperative videoprint above reveals a mass that might have been mistaken for a benign polyp on mirror examination (arrow). There was erythema and fullness anteriorly. Actually, this "polyp" was the tip of a squamous cell carcinoma extending into the supraglottic and infraglottic regions, with cartilage invasion. It involved the true and false vocal folds bilaterally. The tumor was staged $T_4N_0M_0$.

# SECTION IX

# Vocal Fold Trauma

# 68

# Postintubation Vocal Fold Scar

Robert Thayer Sataloff
Mary Hawkshaw
Cheryl A. Hoover
Joseph R. Spiegel

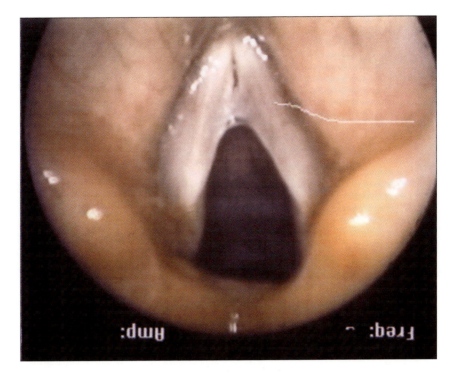

**Fig 68–1**

This 12-year-old girl had a lifetime history of hoarseness. She underwent repair of aortic coarctation at the age of 5 weeks. She presented at this time because she was interested in studying singing and pursuing a performance career. The voice teacher with whom she wanted to study refused to teach her without laryngologic evaluation because of her high, slightly weak and somewhat breathy voice quality. She had seen another otolaryngologist who diagnosed recurrent laryngeal nerve paralysis and "bilateral vocal fold nodules." This patient also admitted to a significant history of gastroesophageal reflux disease beginning at birth, and she reported continued, daily symptoms of reflux.

The videoprint taken during strobovideolaryngoscopy, reveals arytenoid erythema due to laryngopharyngeal reflux and a scar band connecting the two vocal folds. The anterior-most portion of the vocal folds is spared. Therefore, this lesion is a synechia rather than a web. The patient also had left recurrent laryngeal nerve paralysis.

While there was some concern about resecting this scar because of the probability that the attachment between the vocal folds might be helping to overcome the recurrent nerve paralysis, surgery was performed. Both vocal folds healed well, and normal mucosal wave returned. Her fundamental frequency lowered to a normal range, and she experienced no increased problems with glottic closure. Voice therapy and singing lessons have been initiated.

# 69

# Laryngeal Foreign Body in a Former Tracheotomy Patient

Joseph R. Spiegel
Robert Thayer Sataloff
Cheryl A. Hoover

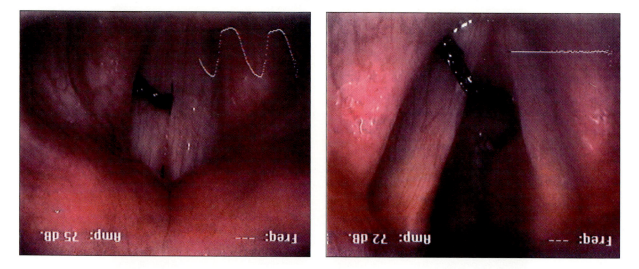

**Fig 69–1**

**Fig 69–2**

This 33-year-old man sustained a head injury on the job in October of 1996 and underwent subsequent tracheotomy. He was decannulated without difficulty 1 month later. He had no complications until 5 months later when he reported a foreign body sensation. He described the sensation as a feeling of "something flipping" in his throat. He was coughing intermittently but was not stridorous, and he denied dysphagia. Strobovideolaryngoscopy revealed a piece of suture originating in the trachea and extending between his vocal folds, preventing complete closure (Figs 69–1 and 69–2). The patient underwent microdirect laryngoscopy and removal of the laryngeal foreign body.

# 70

# Vocal Fold Masses Related to Inhalation of Fumes

Robert Thayer Sataloff
Mary Hawkshaw
Joseph R. Spiegel

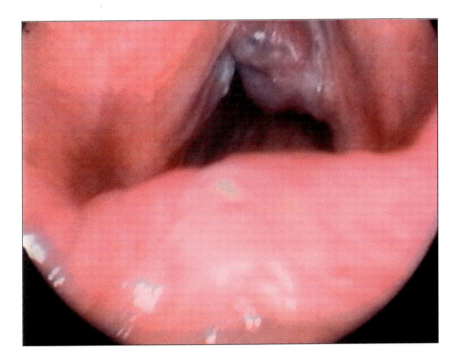

**Fig 70–1**

This 38-year-old man had worked for large rubber and chemical companies for nearly 20 years. His job involved handling malfunctions, including those associated with environmental contamination with fumes. He first developed hoarseness in 1991. Four weeks later, he sustained heavy exposure to vinyl chloride fumes during a reactor malfunction. This incident caused marked, prolonged coughing, and it was serious enough to require his transport to the hospital by ambulance. Within 2 to 3 weeks following this incident, he experienced severe dysphonia. The dysphonia persisted, and the following year he underwent excision of bilateral "vocal fold polyps." His voice improved, but he still had intermittent dysphonia. He returned to work and had no further problems until he was exposed to anhydrous ammonia fumes. Dysphonia recurred and persisted, and was treated with excision of another polyp the following month. His voice improved somewhat, but deteriorated quickly as soon as he returned to work and experienced even minor exposure to fumes. He was also bothered by gasoline fumes when he fueled his car. He had smoked one pack of cigarettes daily from age 16 through 20, quit smoking until he was age 33, then resumed smoking one pack of cigarettes per day. He had quit again at the age of 37. His wife does not smoke, and he is not routinely exposed to secondary smoke. Although he denied dyspepsia, he admitted to a chronic globus sensation. He also stated that his voice was worse in the morning, improved after brief use, and then deteriorated after more extensive phonation. This videoprint was taken during strobovideolaryngoscopy. It revealed an extremely large right vocal fold mass, a small left mass (probably reactive), right vocal fold varicosity (not seen in this videoprint), bilateral vocal fold scarring, muscular tension dysphonia, and gastroesophageal reflux laryngitis. Barium swallow documented hiatal hernia. Pulmonary function tests were at the lower limit of normal. This mass could easily be mistaken for a malignancy. It was removed with traditional instruments, and a laser was used to vaporize the varicosity. Pathology revealed squamous epithelial hyperplasia with organizing hemorrhage and dilated vessels on the right. On the left, there was a hyaline nodule with hemorrhage and cyst formation. Following resection, the patient was restricted from fume exposure. He also received strict antireflux treatment. He did not return to his previous job. His voice remained normal for 2 years until he was accidentally exposed to hydrocarbon fumes. His voice deteriorated immediately and masses recurred, which required excision again. His voice has remained normal for more than 1 year since that procedure, and he has carefully avoided all noxious inhalants.

# 71

# Endolaryngeal Burns From Lye Ingestion

Karen M. Lyons
Robert Thayer Sataloff
Mary Hawkshaw

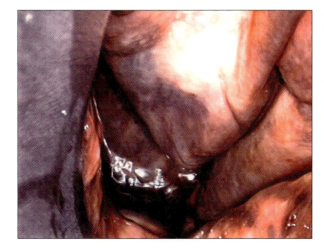

Fig 71–1

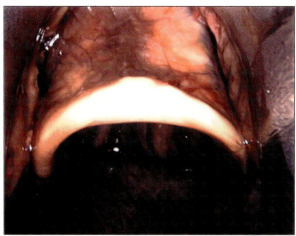

Fig 71–2

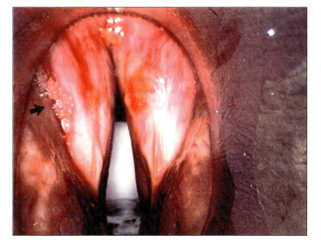

Fig 71–3A

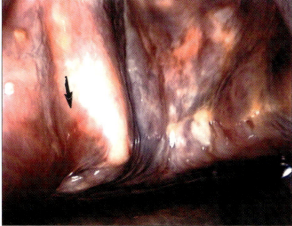

Fig 71–3B

This 59-year-old woman presented to the emergency room awake and alert but vomiting. She had attempted suicide by ingesting lye a few hours prior to her arrival. Within minutes after arriving, she rapidly developed respiratory distress and was intubated by emergency room staff. The author (KML) was consulted promptly to perform microdirect laryngoscopy and tracheotomy in the operating

# 73

# Vocal Fold Avulsion

Robert Thayer Sataloff
Reinhardt J. Heuer
Mary Hawkshaw
Joseph R. Spiegel

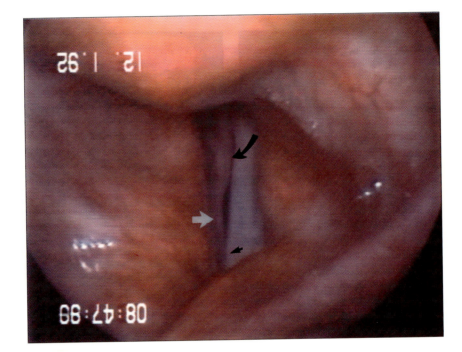

**Fig 73–1**

This 26-year-old man had no voice problems until 5 years prior to examination when he was involved in a motor vehicle accident during which he struck his neck on the steering wheel. Nasotracheal intubation was performed in an emergency room. Laryngeal fracture was diagnosed with a "degloving injury of the left arytenoid." This was repaired by another otolaryngologist through a laryngofissure. The operative note indicated that the mucosa was sutured together. His voice remained extremely hoarse despite voice therapy. Laryngoplasty was performed 8 months later. His voice was stronger for 48 hours but became soft again. Four months later he underwent Teflon injection, which resulted in improvement, but the voice remained extremely soft and hoarse. Teflon injection was repeated 6 months

later without significant change. The voice remained stable during the intervening 3½ years that preceded his referral to Philadelphia. He complained that his voice was soft, breathy, and fatigued easily. He also became hoarse after exercising. His profession required him to speak in a noisy environment, and his vocal dysfunction had become severe enough that he felt it necessary for him to change jobs unless his voice could be improved.

Strobovideolaryngoscopy revealed an unusual combination of findings. His right vocal fold was normal. The left vocal fold was erythematous. Laterally, in the ventricular area (not shown) there was evidence of Teflon granuloma. However, most strikingly, the left vocal process was 3–4 mm below the right vocal process, allowing the right vocal fold to overlap the left during adduction (straight arrow). There was also an area of fullness anteriorly (curved area) and marked mass deficiency posteriorly (white arrow). The anterior fullness was soft, and consequently not due to Teflon in the vibratory margin. Both arytenoids were mobile, but left vocal fold mobility was markedly diminished. The patient had suffered avulsion of his left vocal process, and the thyroarytenoid muscle had contracted anteriorly. These findings were confirmed at the time of laryngofissure. Much of the Teflon was removed, and the vocal process was sutured to the arytenoid at an appropriate height. The voice improved somewhat. However, as expected because of Teflon granuloma and muscle atrophy, it was not possible to restore normal voice.

# 74

# Laryngeal Trauma and Laryngeal Pain

Robert Thayer Sataloff          Mary Hawkshaw
Allyson Shaw                     Karen M. Lyons

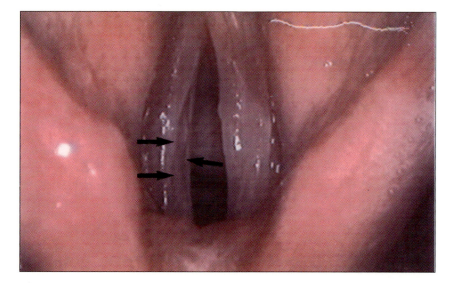

**Fig 74–1.** Videoprint showing diffuse, chronic laryngitis with dark, dusky appearance of both vocal folds. The patient also had posterior laryngeal erythema, edema, and cobblestoning from chronic reflux laryngitis. The small apparent mass on the right vocal fold edge is due to secretions. The groove along the left vocal fold (arrows) is a sulcus. There is stiffness in this area, and the abnormality is believed to be due to trauma and hemorrhage associated with his injury. However, the sulcus is largely below the upper edge of the vibratory margin and does not involve the anterior half of the membranous vocal fold. Consequently, it did not interfere with phonation as much as its appearance may suggest.

This 45-year-old ship's captain was struck on the left side of his neck by a rope that snapped under high tension. The impact raised him 3 feet in the air. He landed on his back, striking the back of his head. He noticed a voice change immediately. He also reported neck pain, dysphagia (greater with liquids than with solids), and a foreign body sensation in his throat.

Direct laryngoscopy, strobovideolaryngoscopy, laryngeal CT, and laryngeal EMG were performed 6 months later. He was found to have a laryngeal fracture involving the left thyroid lamina, profound muscular tension dysphonia, left recurrent laryngeal nerve paresis, right superior laryngeal nerve paresis, reflux laryngitis, and chronic smoking-induced laryngitis (Fig 74-1). His muscular tension dysphonia was secondary to laryngeal pain. He was able to speak with more normal phonation, but was unwilling to do so because of discomfort. His voice could not be restored through voice therapy alone. He underwent thyroplasty to medialize the left vocal fold, and open reduction with internal fixation of his left thyroid cartilage fracture. This resulted in marked improvement in his laryngeal discomfort. Pain relief, along with intensive voice therapy, resulted in elimination of his muscular tension dysphonia and restoration of essentially normal phonation. His reflux laryngitis was controlled with medication and diet, and hypnosis and psychotherapy were used to help him to stop smoking, thus improving his chronic laryngitis. By the time his therapy was completed, he was able to resume avocational singing.

# SECTION X

# Impaired Vocal Fold Mobility

# 75

# Vocal Fold Paralysis

Joseph R. Spiegel
Robert Thayer Sataloff
Mary Hawkshaw

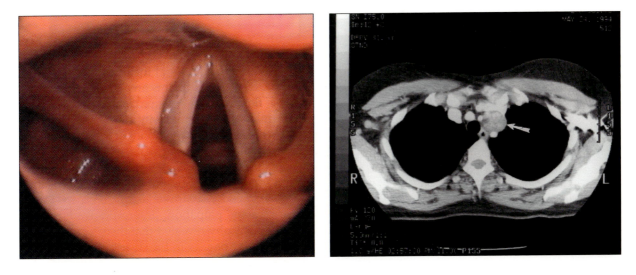

**Fig 75–1.** Left recurrent and superior laryngeal nerve paralysis.

**Fig 75–2.** Schwannoma of the left vagus nerve (arrow).

This 42-year-old teacher had no voice problems until August 1993 when she developed gradually progressive hoarseness, breathiness, decreased volume, and voice fatigue. Her voice was best in the morning, and she was nearly aphonic by the end of her teaching day. Initially, her symptoms were intermittent, but they became persistent over a period of 2 to 3 months.

Physical examination revealed immobility of the left vocal fold. Strobovideolaryngoscopy showed that the vocal processes were approximately at the same level. However, the left vocal fold was ab-ducted, bowed, and flaccid (Fig 75–1). A jostle sign was present (the left arytenoid moved passively when contacted by the right arytenoid). The left vocal fold appeared short, and its longitudinal tension did not increase normally with changes in pitch. Laryngeal electromyography confirmed left recurrent nerve paralysis with marked weakness of the superior laryngeal nerve. Comprehensive evaluation included chest CT, which revealed a left mediastinal mass (Fig 75–2). The diagnosis of vagus nerve schwannoma was confirmed surgically, and the lesion was resected in its entirety through the neck.

## References

1. Sataloff RT, Feldman M, Darby KS, et al. Arytenoid dislocation. *J Voice*. 1988;1:368–377.
2. Sataloff RT, Bough ID, Spiegel JR. Arytenoid dislocation: diagnosis and treatment. *Laryngoscope*. 1994; 104(10):1353–1361.
3. Sataloff RT. *Professional Voice: The Science and Art of Professional Care*. 2nd ed. San Diego, Calif: Singular Publishing Group; 1997:193, 383, 480, 535-537, 639–640.

# 78

# Complex Bilateral Arytenoid Dislocation

Robert Thayer Sataloff
Mary Hawkshaw
Joseph R. Spiegel

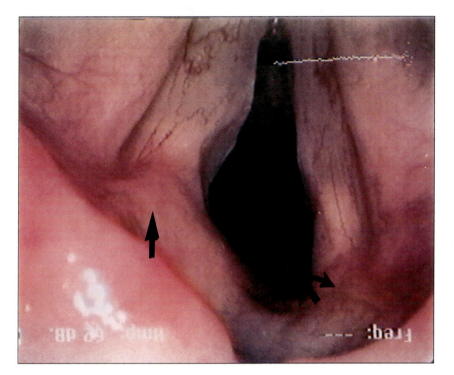

**Fig 78–1**

This 62-year-old teacher was seen in our office for the first time approximately 10 months ago. She was diagnosed 4 years ago with stage II Hodgkins lymphoma and underwent staging laparotomy and splenectomy. She awoke from the operative procedure with a very sore throat, hoarseness, and breathiness. She recalls the nasogastric tube being in place for approximately 1 week after surgery and that removal of this tube was very painful and "somewhat bloody." She stated that the laryngologist who examined her following this surgery diagnosed inflamed vocal folds and treated her with expectorants and antihistamines, which had no effect on her voice. She had quit smoking when her diagnosis of Hodgkins was made after having

smoked at least half a pack of cigarettes a day for 40 years. In her work as an artist and teacher, she reported exposure to multiple inhalants including lead, platinum dust, clay, solvents, and many others. She rarely consumed alcohol. Following her surgery, she was treated with radiation to her left neck and chest. She developed severe shortness of breath during radiation therapy. Bronchoscopy was performed and she was treated with Prednisone, which helped her breathing but not her voice.

One year prior to her first office visit with us, she was found to have a left sublingual lymph node that was non-Hodgkins lymphoma. She was treated with 6 cycles of chemotherapy that were completed 4 months after the diagnosis. Her metatastic workup was negative. She developed hypothyroidism following this treatment. Her voice remained breathy, and she had inspiratory stridor when we first examined her.

Strobovideolaryngoscopy revealed bilateral vocal fold immobility and very unusual posturing of the arytenoids. The arytenoids were at different heights, and it appeared as if the right arytenoid (curved arrow; Fig 78–1) was dislocated posteriorly and the left arytenoid (straight arrow) was dislocated anteriorly. There was distortion in her posterior arytenoid region, as well. She was evaluated further by 3D CT scan of the larynx, MRI of the brain to the level of the mediastinum, laryngeal EMG, voice therapy, and pulmonary function tests, as well as barium swallow. One month later she was taken to the operating room where micro-direct laryngoscopy was performed. Interoperatively, the left vocal fold was found to be displaced posteriorly, medially, and inferiorly. Her voice improved following surgery, and her airway was adequate. The right arytenoid was not manipulated at the time of this surgery to prevent airway obstruction, but it may require surgery in the future.

# 79

# Autologous Fat Injection: The Intraoperative End Point

Robert Thayer Sataloff
Mary Hawkshaw
Allyson Shaw

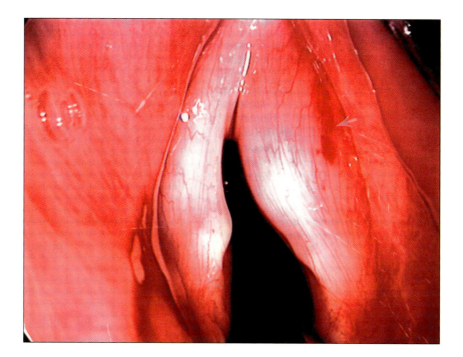

**Fig 79–1**

This patient was a 40-year-old marketing executive and avocational performer of musical theater. He was active in choral performance as a youth and had several years of vocal training during that time, but none since. Approximately 1 year prior to our evaluation, he noticed hoarseness, decreased range, dryness, breathiness, and a general sense that "my cords aren't working right." His diagnostic evaluation included strobovideolaryngoscopy, laryngeal EMG, blood tests, and imaging studies. He was found to have right vocal fold paresis, presumably as a consequence of Lyme disease. He could not compensate for his glottic incompetence through voice and singing therapy alone. He was taken to the operating room for autologous fat injection. The intraoperative figure shows 30% to 40% overcorrection following injection at one location laterally (arrow). There is a small superficial hematoma adjacent to the injection site. The apparent bowing of the left vocal fold is artifact.

3  5282  00553  5417